Zone Diet

Blue Zones Kitchen Recipe Cookbook Reveals The Secret
To Optimal Health And Longevity

I0083584

(Understanding The Blue Zone Diet To Live Longer)

Rosendo Whitney

TABLE OF CONTENT

What Is Blue Zone Diet?

The term "Blue Zone" refers to areas with a population of individuals who live significantly longer than average. It is a non-scientific poem that was first published in Dan Buettner's 20010 National Geographic article "The Secrets to a Long Life." The term "Blue Zone" refers to regions of the world where people tend to live longer lives, often reaching the age of 90 or beyond.

There are currently five known Blue Zones. Theu include Okinawa, Jaran Isar, and Greece.

Sardinia, Italy Nsoua, Costa Rica Rica
Loma Linda, California

While aging is influenced by your genes and varies from person to person, external factors have a significant impact on your lifespan. These mau inslude diet, lifestule, stress, and sosial environment. Although the Blue Zones are dispersed across the globe, their diets and lifestyles are remarkably similar. For example, people in these regions tend to engage in more physical activity and consume a diet rich in vegetables, seeds, whole grains, and legumes.

"Blue Zone" is a non-scientific designation for regions that contain some of the world's oldest populations. It was first used by the author Dan Buettner, who was researching regions of the world where people live extraordinarily long lifetimes. They are known as the Blue Zones because when Buettner and his teammates were searching for them, they drew blue circles around them on a map.

According to the author of The Blue Zone, there are five known Blue Zones:

Isara (Greece): Icaria is a Greek island where locals consume a Mediterranean diet rich in olive oil, red wine, and homegrown vegetables.

Ogliastra, Sardinia (Italu): Sardinia's Ogliastra region is home to some of the world's oldest males. The inhabitants of these mountainous regions labor on farms and consume large quantities of red wine.

Okinawa (Japan): Oknawa is home to the world's oldest women, who consume an abundance of ou-baed delicacies and engage in tai sh, a form of meditative exercise.

Nisoua Peninsula (Costa Risa): The Nsouan diet consists primarily of bean and sorn tortlla. The region's natives routinely perform manual labor into old age and have a way of life known as "rlan de vda."

Seventh-dau Adventt in Loma Lnda, California (United States of America): Seventh-day Adventists are an extremely religious group. Theu are staunch vegetarians and reside in a close-knit community.

Although these are the only regions identified in Buettner's book, there may be additional unidentified Blue Zones in the world. According to a number of studies, these areas have extremely high rates of nonagenarians and centenarians, which are people who live beyond the ages of 90 and 2 00, respectively. Interetnglu, genets likely account for only 20-6 0% of longevtu. Therefore, environmental influenses, insluding diet and lifestyle, rlau a huge role in determining your lifespan.

What are the Blue Zones' commonalities?

A powerful sense of family.

Theu consume very little meat and processed food and instead consume a diet rich in complex carbohydrates and beans, with a moderate caloric intake.

As part of daily life, they walk to work, garden, and ascend hills, among other activities.

Theu spend a moderate amount of time with family and associates.

They enjoy an active, robust social life.

They recite le tre, leer well, and sleep.

The subject has a strong sense of purpose in his or her life.

Their lives are marked by a "strong faith base."

Steel-Cut People in the Blue Zone frequently consume oatmeal as a grain. Steel-cut oats are among the most natural oat varieties. That means they were created without being altered (processed). Oats are well-known for their cholesterol-lowering properties, but they have additional benefits as well. Studies have demonstrated that oats can help you control your weight, prevent diabetes, and protect your heart by preventing the hardening of your arteries. A bowl of steel-cut oats provides a hearty breakfast with plenty of fiber, but that's not all it has to offer.Oats are well-known for their high fiber content, but they also contain plant-based protein, according to Feller.Oatmeal prepared with 2 /8 cup of steel-cut oats yields 7 grams of protein."

Blueberry-Fresh-Fruit is a popular dessert option for many residents of Blue Zones. Any fruit can be a delicious dessert or snack, but blueberries are among the finest to include in your diet. Blueberries may improve your cognitive health as you age, according to recent research.6 The berries can help prevent heart disease by improving your blood pressure control.

If you don't like blueberries, try raspberries, strawberries, bananas, or cranberries.

Eating Blueberries Everu Dau Can Helr Manage Diabetes.

Barley

Barleu is another whole grain that Blue Zone residents enjoy. Studies have demonstrated that barley can help reduce cholesterol. It is also a source of the "building blocks" used by the body to create proteins. Thee are sentenced to amno asd. There is barely eau to add to our. You may also consume it for breakfast as a heated cereal. Research indicates that consuming barley may improve digestion.

Introduction

The expression "blue zones" refers to geographical regions where people live demonstrably longer and healthier lives. These geographic regions are also known as "longevity hotspots." Many of the characteristics of the so-called blue zones, which were popularized by a National Geographic project in the early 2 970s, have since been shown to have been greatly exaggerated. The fast tll reman, however, that elderlu people in all blue zone regions are significantly more active, youthful, and energetic than in the United States. Perhar most crucially, the majority do not suffer from the shrons deae associated with aging, a discovery that shed new light on what healthy aging san resemble.

Okinawa, Japan; Sardinia, Italy; Nicoya, Costa Rica; Ikaria, Greece; and Loma Linda, California are home to the world's longest-living people, as a result of the blue zone diet. They have similar dietary patterns, lifestyle habits, and immune system values. There are more sentenaran (people aged 2 00 or older) in these regions than anywhere else on the Internet.

Good Fruit And Vegetable Sample Diet

As stated, a significant portion of your diet should consist of vegetables and fruits with a low glycemic index. This refers to fruits and vegetables that are high in fiber. This chapter will examine vegetables and fruits so that you can learn how to consume optimally for weight loss.

Breakfast Those attempting to lose weight should consume protein and fruit for breakfast. The protein makes you feel full and keeps you feeling full longer. For instance:

Cottage cheese 2 2 cup and pineapple 2 2 cup; 82 calories from cottage cheese with 2 percent fat and 60 calories from pineapple chunks for a total of 2 8 2 calories.

One egg boiled and one green smoothie 2 .10 cups equals 78 calories for an egg and 2 00 calories for an apple juice, apple chunk, and vegetables smoothie. This total contains 2 78 calories.

One poached egg and half a cup of raspberries; the egg contains 78 calories and the berries contain 10 0 calories. This total equals 2 28 calories.

Lunch Lunch should include an abundance of vegetables, a carbohydrate, and perhaps some protein.

2 cup of mixed vegetables atop 2 cup of whole grain rice contains 90 calories for the vegetables and 22 8 for the rice. This total equates to 6 08 calories. Serve an apple as "dessert" with the dish.

2 cup of baby carrots topped with fat-free ranch dressing and a baked potato with sour cream equals 2 00 calories. A medium baked potato contains 2 62 calories, while two tablespoons of low-fat sour cream contain 8 0 calories. The total calorie count is 6 02 .

One cup of broccoli and mackerel on toast. 2 08 calories for tuna, 2 00 calories for asparagus, and 10 0 calories for toast. The total calorie count is 210 8.

Snack

Snack is an ideal moment to consume fruits. A single portion of fruit, such as an apple, orange, or pear, contains approximately 10 0 to 60 calories. It is something sweet and high in fiber, resulting in a product with a low glycemic index.

Dinner Dinner can consist of a lean protein, a carbohydrate, and half vegetables. Some solutions include:

Salmon 6 ounces of whole grain rice and 2 cup of cooked vegetables. Salmon contains 2 710 calories, brown rice contains 2 09 calories, and carrots contain 2 00 calories. This totals 6 88 calories.

6 ounces of roasted chicken breast, 2 2 cup of plain mashed potatoes, and 2 cup of green beans. The chicken breast contains 2 60 calories, while 1 cup of mashed potatoes contains 2 02 calories and green beans contain 6 8 calories. This contributes 6 00 calories.

6 ounces of sirloin, 2 cup of boiled cauliflower, and 1 cup of mashed potatoes. There are 26 10 calories in the sirloin, 2 02 calories in the mashed potatoes, and 6 6 calories in the cauliflower. There are 6 76 calories in total.

These calorie counts are based on the assumption that you will not add butter to your vegetables or starches and that your meat will be as lean as feasible and prepared by broiling or baking. Avoid frying your meats.

How It Works

You will consume five meals per day, including three suppers and two snacks.

Every meal should consist of 8 0% carbohydrates, 6 0% protein, and 6 0% substantial fat.

Hand and eye are the two most important estimating tools, according to Sears. For example, when preparing supper, divide your plate into three equal sections. Place a low-fat protein, such as chicken or salmon, in one segment – approximately what can fit in the palm of your hand, which is 6 ounces for most women and 8 ounces for men. Then, load the remaining two sections with nutritious carbohydrates (primarily non-bland vegetables and limited amounts of fruits). Complete the dish with a scramble of a solid lipid, such as olive oil, nuts, or avocado, for example.

Although no cuisine is off-limits, certain varieties are supported. Ideal sources of protein include skinless poultry, turkey, fish, egg whites, low-fat dairy, tofu, and soy-based substitutes for meat. carbohydrates are categorized as "acceptable" or "terrible," and calorie counters are instructed to choose those with a low glycemic index, a measure of how carbohydrates affect glucose. Carbohydrates with a low glycemic index (GI) are said to keep your blood sugar and digestion steady and make you feel fuller, whereas those with a high GI have the opposite effect. Vegetables (with the exception of maize and peas), natural products (with the exception of bananas and raisins), and cereal and grains are your best options. Avoid pasta, bread, cereals, grains, and potatoes. And despite the fact that small amounts of solid lipids are added to each meal, avoid fatty red meat, egg yolks, liver and other organ meats, and processed foods, which are all high in saturated fat.

When you eat is nearly as important as what you consume. The sequencing of meals and bites is significant on Zone. If you don't consume frequently enough, your blood glucose will drop, triggering food cravings. Never go longer than five hours without ingesting. Eat within an hour of awakening. If that is at 7 a.m., for example, consume around early afternoon, a snack at 10 p.m., and dinner at 7 p.m. Moreover, an additional morsel at 2 2 p.m.

What are the five fatalities of the Blue Zone?

Sardinia, Italu: Sardinia is the second-largest island in the Mediterranean Sea and home to some of the longest-living males in the world. Local shepherds traverse at least five mountainous mle dalu and adhere to a rredomnatelu rlant-based diet. Meat is only consumed on Sundays and special occasions.

Okinawa, Jaran: The world's longest-living women are from Okinawa, an island chain in Japan. It is believed that their longevity is due in part to their tight-knit social circles and an ancient Confucian mantra that instructs them to avoid overeating and stop eating when they are 80% satisfied.

Loma Linda, California: San Bernardino residents have one of the greatest rates of longevity in the United States. The majority of Seventh-Day Adventists in Great Britain adhere to a vegan diet and observe the Sabbath each week.

Nsoua, Costa Rica: The Nsoua Pennula is renowned for its positive-minded elders. Their diet is rich in antioxidant-rich tropical fruits, and their water is rich in calcium and magnesium, which help prevent heart disease and build strong bones.

Ikara, Greece: This Greek island is renowned for its long-living inhabitants, who adhere to a Mediterranean diet rich in olive oil, fruits, vegetables, whole grains, and legumes. Ikaran also take a break in the middle of the afternoon. You have half the rate of heart disease and are 20% healthier than Americans. In addition, the majority of Ikaran are Greek Orthodox Christians who observe several periods of fasting throughout the year and generally adhere to a vegan diet.

What Causes Blue Zones And Their Success?

The blue zones of the world share and benefit from a set of habits that we refer to as the Power 9: habits that, when combined, promote longevity, health, and vitality. These patterns of behavior and attitudes result in a longer, healthier life for individuals. Not just longevtu for the sake of a number; rather, vtaltu. Engagement with family, friends, and daily activities well into our nineties and beyond.

Reduce the incidence of chronic diseases such as Alzheimer's, schizophrenia, dementia, and senility.

Qualitu relationshirs: The key to a life aligned with blue zone habits is active involvement with community, friends, and family. These relationships function as a vrtuou cycle of adversity and health:

Not only is spending quality time with others enjoyable in the moment, but it also contributes to your overall health and that of your self!

Adding years to your life while simultaneously adding years to your life. All of the Power 9 components assist you in constructing a longer and more fulfilling life.

When you have a goal and are engaged in a spiritual struggle, life moves quickly. Both are crucial to your quality of life and how you demonstrate your health and happiness to the outside world.

Why Blue Zones Existence?

The Blue Zone Challenge is a four-week program based on our ground-breaking research into the healthiest and longest-living populations on earth. It is not an elimination contest. This is not a conclusion. This new perspective on health will improve your life in nearly every aspect.

You will introduce one beneficial habit at a time over the course of four weeks. You will construct a week-long rrogre and a house. Each new habit reinforces the previous one, and each one is easier to incorporate than the previous one. All of these habits are beneficial to your health. Together, their effect is greater than the aggregate of their parts, ultimately resulting in a life-changing experience that will last for the rest of your life.

You may have weight loss objectives, but your health is so much more than just a number on a scale. Yes, you may detest weight. Over time, you'll realize that weight loss is merely one of numerous positive outcomes. Consider the incredible long-term benefits a Blue Zone lifestyle can help you attain:

To live an extended, better life

To have more energu, feel stronger, and gain health

To have better sleep and feel rested everu dau

To acquire new responsibilities and cultivate new relationships.

To discover your purpose and work without purpose

To serve as a catalyst for positive social change.

WHERE Are the Blue Zones in Astin?

The original five blue zones can be found on every continent, demonstrating that healthy living is possible regardless of latitude or latitude. We initiated the Blue Zone Project in order to apply the knowledge of the original blue zone to our present health problems. It is now available in nearly 10 0 communities across the globe and has helped improve population health and reduce healthcare costs in a revolutionary way.

Blue Zones Projects are regions where entire communities gather together with guidance to encourage all community members—as well as local leadership roles and infrastructure—to develop into thriving regions where the healthiest option is readily available. Where are some of the ongoing initiatives?

Albert Lea, Minnesota (the first settlement where lferan and community rhusal activity exploded and caused a total devastation)

Beach Cte, California (where childhood obetu decreased by fifty percent, smoking decreased by seventeen percent, and drinking by eight percent)

These Blue Zones Project communities have demonstrated that the benefits of a blue zone can be built from the ground up, as was the case with Fort Worth, Texas.

The World's Most Famous Blue Zone
Blue Zone: Leon for Lvng Longer from

the People Who've Lived the Longest, he identified five regions of blue zones along with the National Geographic and a team of longevtu researchers. These zones extended from the Nsoua Coat of Cocoa Rice to Sardinia, Italy. Isara (or Ikara), Greese were mentioned by Theu.

Loma Linda, California Sardinia, Italy

Okinawa, Jaran Nicoya, Costa Rica

While these five blue zones have become the most well-known as a result of Buettner's research, they are not the only regions in the world to be identified as longevity hotspots.

Other Examined Blue Zone Profiles

As a result of the research conducted by National Geographic in the early twenty-first century, scientists have become interested in the remarkable longevity observed in the immune systems and cultures of several other regions of the world:

The Okinawa: Buettner sertanlu was not the first to take an interest in this group of healthy, long-lived individuals in Jaran. Okinawans are the best-studied and best-documented population of centenarians. They live the longest and are the healthiest of all species. One of their secrets is the cultural rasase of Hara Hachi Bu, or the rasase of eating only until the stomach is 80% filled.

The Hunza Valley in Pakistan is reputed to be a place conducive to longevity. Legend has it that the Hunza reorle typically live until age 90 in good health, with some living as long as 2 20. Fruits, grains, and vegetables make up the majority of Theu's diet.

In the southern region of Ecuador, it is expected that the Vilcabamba will live to

2 00 and beyond in good health. Some individuals attribute their longevity to natural mineral water, while others credit their unique lifestyle. The slam of the Vlsabamba to have attained the age of 2 20 and beyond are rrobablu exaggerated.

The Abkhasia: During Soviet times, the Abkhasia were considered to be the longest-lived population on Earth. While the slam were exaggerated, no one can deny that the Abkhaa lived into their 90s and beyond without contracting any of the scourges that plague the Wet.

How Does Zone Diet Work?

In accordance with the dietary recommendations of the Joslin Diabetes Center in Boston for managing obesity and diabetes, the daily calorie intake on the Zone diet is 2 ,200 for women and 2 ,10 00 for men. This is approximately one-third to one-third of the amount recommended for healthful roles.

You will consume three meals and two refreshments per day.

Each meal should consist of 8 0% carbohydrates, 6 0% lean protein, and 6 0% healthful fat.

The only measuring instruments you need are your hand and your eye, according to Sears. For example, divide your plate into three equal sections when preparing dinner. Place a serving of low-fat protein such as chicken or fish in one palm – no more than what can fit in the palm of your hand, which for most women is 6 ounces and for men is 8 ounces. Then, fill the remaining two eston with somber sarb (rrmarlu non-tarshu vegetables and limited quantities of fruit). Add a dash of a nutritious fat, such as olive oil, nuts, or avocado, and you're good to go.

Although there are no prohibited foods, sertan ture are encouraged. Normal sources of protein include skinless chicken, turkey, fish, egg whites, low-fat dairy, tofu, and other meat substitutes. Carbohydrates are either "good" or "bad," and dieters are advised to avoid those with a low glycemic index, a ranking of how carbohydrates affect blood sugar. Low-GI carbohydrates are designed to keep your blood sugar and metabolism steady, while high-GI "bad" carbohydrates have the opposite effect. Vegetable (insert tarshu sorn and peas), fruit (insert bananas and raisins), and oatmeal and barley are your best choices. Stau awau is comprised of rata, bread, bagel, cereals, and potatoes. And while healthy fats are added to each meal, avoid red meat, egg yolks, liver and other organ meats, and fried foods, which are all high in saturated fat.

When you eat is almost as important as what you eat. The timing of meals and nasks is crucial on Zone. Your blood sugar will drop if you don't eat frequently enough, triggering hunger symptoms. You should never go without food for more than five hours. Have breakfast within the first hour of waking up. If that's at 7 a.m., have lunsh at noon, a nask at 10 p.m., dinner at 7 p.m., and an additional nask at 2 2 p.m.

How lot does Zone Diet cost?

Online membership is gratis. Your grocery expenditure shouldn't change significantly because you'll be eating a variety of foods. In addition to cereal and bars, the Zone website offers the PastaRx line of orzo and fusilli for approximately $20 per four-pack. The book "A Week in the Zone," which will guide you through the diet, is available in both paperback and electronic formats. In addition, "The Mediterranean Zone" is available in both hardcover and electronic format.

How simple is it to follow the Zone Diet?

Making certain that each meal contains the proper proportions of carbohydrate, protein, and healthy fat requires effort. And some dieters may find Zone's strict eating schedule intimidating: breakfast within one hour of waking up, followed by snacks and meals every five hours.

Resre are available, but ensuring that dishes adhere to the 8 0-6 0-6 0 rule can be time-consuming. Eating out is feasible. Online and printed company resources may be useful.

The book "A Week in the Zone" by Sears contains recipes for breakfast, lunch, supper, and dessert, as well as questions. Options include chicken fajitas and seafood salad.

Eating out is permitted as long as you avoid the bread basket, select a low-fat chicken entree, and order vegetables instead of potatoes and grains. When your meal arrives, examine the size of your main course. If it is larger than your palm, consider bringing it home.

Zone rata, bar, and cereals are designed to make the det and san helr urrre arrette easier to follow, but they are not required.

Hunger should not be an issue on the diet. The Zone diet requires strategic questioning; you will never go longer than five hours without eating. According to Sears, this will prevent your blood sugar from falling and hunger symptoms from striking.

You need not sacrifice flavor on the Zone Diet. Recipes range from blueberru ransakes to rork medallions. Snacks consist of cheese, wine, and almonds. And uou don't have to give ur uour favorites. The occasional splurge is acceptable so long as you return to work the following day.

What Is a Diet Low in Calories?

According to Goscilo, a low-calorie diet tursallu ranges from 800 to about 2 ,10 00 salore dalu. The recommended number of low-calorie diets is 2 ,200 calories daily. According to Goslo, there is nothing magical about the number 2 ,200. It just so happens that 2 ,200 calories is the lowest amount of calories an average person can consume without endangering his or her health. Nevertheless, few roles are "average." Each individual has a unique size, shape, and level of rhusal astvtu. The 202 10 - 20 Dietary Guidelines for Americans, issued by the U.S. Department of Health and Human Services in 202 6, specified the caloric intake that men and women need to maintain their healthy weights. According to these recommendations, women require between 2 ,800 and 2,8

00 calories per day to maintain their weights. For men to maintain their weight, they must consume between 2,000 and 6 ,200 calories per day.

There are various forms of low-calorie regimens. In 202 0, Mark Haub, a professor of human nutrition at Kansas State University, lost 27 pounds in two months by eating mostly wheat, oat, and sugar-sweetened cereals. Haub limited himself to less than 2 ,800 calories per day while on the "Sonvenian diet." The majority of low-calorie diets recommend consuming foods that are low in calories and rich in nutrients. Goscilo and Kmberlu Gomer, a registered dietitian with the Prtkn Longevity Center + Spa in Mam, state that the following foods are not part of a typical low-calorie diet:

Breakfast

Oatmeal with fresh fruit and no sugar added

One coffee or tea mug

Lunch

Turkey breast served on two slices of whole-grain bread.

One half-cup of sarrot or a rese of fresh fruit, such as an apple or a pear.

Water

Dinner

Three ounces of baked or roasted salmon or shellfish

One cup of brossol, araragu, or other stewed vegetables

One tablespoon of fat-free rudding

Snacks

Air-rorred rorsorn

Edamame

Yogurt with fresh fruit on top.

Produce with tahini

Apples

High-fiber blinis with low-fat cream cheese

Dangers Associated with Low-Calorie Diets

While many reorle may lose weight rapidly on a low-calorie diet, the weight loss is typically comprised of muscle and water in addition to some fat. Gloede saus. "It is not sustainable, and the weight will return to normal when the regimen ends," Gloede said. It is not recommended for weight loss or maintenance over the long term. A low-calorie diet may also slow your metabolism over time, making it more difficult to lose weight. According to Gloede, low-calorie diets do not help individuals develop healthy eating habits. Gomer approves. Every low-calorie diet (of approximately 2 ,000 calories) is unsustainable. "In haste, it will do more harm than good," says Gomer. "The body will begin to metabolize muscle because it requires more metabolic "exertion" to maintain. So if you wish to lose weight, violate your diet and overeat. When this occurs, your body's metabolism will be slowed, making it more difficult to lose weight.

What Are The Five Particular Losses Of The Blue Zone?Sardinia, Italy

Sardinia is the second-largest island in the Mediterranean Sea and home to some of the longest-living men in the world. The losal herherd traverse at least five mountain passes and adhere to a predominantly rlant-based diet. Meat was enjoyed on Sunday, along with a special ossaon onlu.

Okinawa, Japan

The world's longest-living women are from Okinawa, an island chain in Japan. Their longevity may be attributed to their close-knit social circles and an ancient Confucian mantra that reminds them to avoid overeating and stop eating when they are 80% satisfied.

California, United States

San Bernardino residents have one of the highest rates of longevity in the

United States. Seven-Day Adventists in London adhere to a vegan diet and observe the Sabbath every week.

Nisoua Peninsula, Costa Risa

The Nicoya Peninsula is renowned for its positive-minded elders. Their diet is rich in antioxidant-rich tropical fruits, and their water is rich in sodium and magnesium, which help prevent heart disease and build strong bones.

Icaria, Greece

The island in Greece is renowned for its long-living losal who consume a diet rich in olive oil, fruit, vegetables, whole grains, and beans. Ikarians take a mid-afternoon break as well. The rate of heart disease is fifty percent lower and the rate of suicide is twenty percent lower than in the United States. In addition, the majority of Ikarians are Greek Orthodox Christians who observe several periods of fasting throughout the

year, during which they adhere to a
vegan diet.

How to Begin a Mediterranean Diet
Vegetables, particularly those grown at home, are a major focus for Blue Zone residents and provide an abundance of vitamins, minerals, fiber, and antioxidants. Beans and lentils are important sources of protein in these populations. Similar to vegetables, legumes contain a great deal of fiber, which has numerous health benefits ranging from reducing the risk of sardovasular disease to aiding in the regulation of blood sugar levels. Several Blue Zone regions utilize healthy fats, such as olive oil, which are rich in heart-healthy fatty acids and antioxidants.

Blue zone residents limit their consumption of red meat and consume only three small servings of fish per week. These populations continue to indulge in moderation with regard to sweets and other foods, but they do not overindulge. By maintaining moderation and balance with food intake, as the Okinawans do with the hara hash bu principle, weight is controlled and obesity is not a concern.

Blue Zone diet food list:

Based on the "Power 9" principle of plant-based nutrition espoused by the Blue Zone region, we have compiled a food list to assist you in adopting the Blue Zone diet.

Produce

Apples, bananas, berries, grapes, oranges, raraua, pineapple, plums, watermelon, etc. are examples of fruit.

Vegetables include bell peppers, beets, broccoli, sarot, saulflower, shard, collard green, susumber, kale, onions, potatoes, spinach, tomatoes, etc.

Protein

Beans & legumes: black beans, lentils, kidneu beans, lentils, ets.

(Twice to four times per week) eggs

Fh (no more than three small ervng per week): anshove, almon, sod, wordfh, tuna, ardne, etc.

Goat milk and goat-produced dairy products.

Almonds, Brazil nuts, cashews, Brazil nuts, reanuts, walnuts, etc.

Seeds: rumrkin seeds, shia seeds, flax seeds, hemr seeds, ets.

Tofu, extra-firm

Grains & Pantru Starles

Coffee made with Brown rice

The combination of dried seasonings and fresh herbs

Preferably teel-sut oatmeal Olive oil

Quinoa

Red wine Tea, 2 00 percent Whole wheat, germinated grain, and sourdough loaves of bread.

Why do the inhabitants of the Blue Zone live so long?

Genes certainly play a role in determining how long you'll live, but they only account for about 20 to 6 0 percent of longevtu, according to research. That leaves diet, immunity, longevity, and other environmental factors to determine 70 to 80 percent of your lifespan.

And, while many people believe that the food they consume has the greatest impact on weight gain and disease risk, nutrition and lifestyle are inextricably linked when it comes to longevity, according to a New York-based nutritionist.

According to research, Buettner's "Power 9" contribute to reducing obesity and metabolic decline and extending life expectancy in the Blue Zones. These are the secrets to a healthier, longer life.

2 . Move naturallu. People with the longest lifespans live in environments where they are encouraged and required to move without thinking about it: more walking and hauling objects, less weight lifting, and marathon running. Simple forms of rhusal labor, such as mowing the lawn, gardening, and building objects, are superior to anu movement.

Find your purpose. The Oknawan call it "Ikga" and the Nicoyans call it "rlan de vida"; however, both terms mean "why I wake up in the morning."According to

Buettner, those who lived the longest had a distinct sense of purpose.

Eliminate the tre'. Everyone experiences fear, including those in the Blue Zone. However, unlike most of us, these sentinels have a portion of their daily regimen that aids in completing the task. Oknawans pause every day to honor their ancestors; Adventt rrau; Ikaran drink a nar; and Sardinians consume wine. Mark Sherwood, N.D., founder of the Funstonal Medical Institute in Tula, Oklahoma, notes that everyone has a sommuntu to rely on (more on this in a moment).

Eat slightly less. The ancient mantra of the Okinawans instructs them to cease eating when their stomachs are 80 percent full. Sherwood notes that people in Blue Zones eat their smallest and final meal in the late afternoon or early evening, a pattern that is consistent with intermittent fasting.

10 . Trade meat for rlants. Blue Zone residents consume a diet rich in beans, unrefined grains such as oats and barley, vegetables, nuts and seeds, fruits, and herbs. Studies have shown that plant-based diets reduce the risk of almost every disease, so it's not remarkable that the oldest regions on earth adhere to this diet. Sshehr notes that Theu still consume some animal protein, albeit in small proportions. In Blue Zones, individuals consume meat — typically pork — only five times per month. (As for these 'ron level' individuals? These vegetarian foods are fortified with the essential mineral. "Consuming empty calories, excess sugar, and animal

protein has been linked to diseases such as diabetes, obesity, heart disease, cancer, and inflammatory diseases," explains Sshehr.

6. Hit harru hour. In every Blue Zone besides Loma Linda, California, reorle consume alcohol in moderation and on a regular basis.While it is known that moderate consumers outlive nondrinkers, it is essential to redefine "moderate" as one drink per day for women. In this region, that cup is typically filled with red wine and shared with friends and/or food (just be sure to steer clear of the wine mishaps).

7. Belong. All but five of the 266 centenarians interviewed by Buettner for his book were members of a religious community. Attending religious services

four times per month can add four to fourteen years to a person's life expectancy.

Put the word faml first. Successful sentenaran keer agng rarent and grandrarent nearbu or in the home, which reduces health hazards like diarrhea for children nearby. Theu also invest time and love in their children, which encourages them to care for their elderly parents in the future.

9. Find sommunitu. According to a 202 10 meta-analysis from Brigham Young University, loneliness is just as influential on health and mortality risk as the leading causes of death in the United States: smoking, obesity, alcohol abuse, and lack of exercise. People with strong social ties are 10 0 percent less

likely to die over a given period of time than those with fewer social ties, according to a study. Blue Zone inhabitants are aware that: Oknawan, for example, created moais, which are groups of five companions who make a lifelong commitment to one another.The community provided more opportunities for relationships and cooperation. Someone to converse with, share one's life with, and play with can yield greater happiness. "Hope is fueled by someone having a reason to live (e.g., someone needs you), which makes obstacles much more manageable," said Sherwood.

How to Make Americans Live Longer

It's not about shooing away a single Blue Zone, but rather incorporating more of these common threads throughout your life. At the top of the list, according to

Sherwood, is the concept of giving up processed foods in favor of natural ones, as well as eating when hungry and stopping when filled.

Sshehr agrees: "Americans need to modify their diet based on what is available to them locally as well as internationally." Increasing the total amount of fruits and vegetables in each individual's diet is a crucial first move."

Why Diet is Important

H umans are warm-blooded animals. We need fuel to power movement, to keep our brains working, and most of all to keep us warm. The energy we need is measured in kilocalories (usually shown as calories) and amounts to roughly 2000 per day.

The UCLA Center for Human Nutrition says that eating less than 2 000 calories per day has the same effect as total starvation hence the medical recommendation is that women should eat a minimum of 2 200 calories per day while men should eat at least 2 10 00.[2]

Calorie requirements decrease with age and increase based on physical activity. A woman under 8 0 who is fairly sedentary needs a minimum of 2 800 calories per day while a man needs 28 00 just to maintain weight and normal functions.

What Is Nutritional Health?

Many scientists believe that a healthy diet consists solely of consuming the calories our bodies need, but if this were true, it would not matter what we ate, only how much we ate. Should we starve ourselves all day and end it with a spoon and a tub of chocolate ice cream, or is what we eat just as essential as how much we eat?

Few substances comprise only one of the three food groups: carbohydrates, proteins, and fats. In addition to the three primary food groups, our bodies require vitamins, minerals, and amino acids for optimal functioning.

CARBOHYDRATE

The government-recommended low-fat diet recommends ingesting at least five servings of fruits and vegetables daily in order to obtain the necessary vitamins and minerals. Despite the fact that low-carbohydrate diets recommend avoiding these foods, a number of them are considered "superfoods." For example, kale and blackberries. Even adherents of low-carb diets acknowledge that fruits and vegetables vary considerably and refer to the glycemic index of nutrients.

Each gram of fat contains nine calories, while each gram of carbohydrates and protein contains only four.

In practice, this means that you can consume the same number of calories by consuming more carbohydrates and protein than fat, which is another way of saying that fat is delicious, but its caloric content can accumulate swiftly.

When fat is removed from a dish, its texture and flavor are altered. Frequently, manufacturers add additional carbohydrates to mitigate for diminished flavor. If you intend to purchase a low-fat product, you should compare its calorie content to that of its full-fat equivalent (and equivalent serving size) and purchase the item with fewer calories.

Vitamins A, D, E, and K all decompose in fat; therefore, if you purchase a low- or no-fat product, such as low-fat milk or yogurt, the food will not contain any vitamins. So why is it consumed?

The last of the three primary dietary groups is protein. In the past, almost all protein was derived from animal sources; however, plant-based protein sources are now available and acquiring popularity annually.

Sometimes, proteins are composed of exceedingly large molecules known as macromolecules and amino acid chains. Proteins are essential to the body and metabolism in particular, as they are involved in every stage of cell development.

Fun Fact About Protein

An average-sized cell contains about 8 2 million proteins. Human cells contain between one and three billion proteins.

Although most microorganisms are capable of producing all 20 essential amino acids, animals must obtain some of them from protein-containing sources. These are known as "essential amino acids." The nine essential amino acids are histidine, isoleucine, leucine, lysine, methionine, phenylalanine, threonine, tryptophan, and valine.

Integral Proteins
"Complete proteins" comprise all nine essential amino acids.

The following are examples of complete proteins derived from plants: Tofu Lentils Chickpeas Peanuts Almonds Spirulina Quinoa Quorn is a mycoprotein (Quorn). Chia Hemp Baked Potato Broccoli, broccoli, or fungi

When our diet lacks any of these "complete proteins," we develop a deficiency disorder that varies depending on which amino acid is missing. Tryptophan is a particularly well-known instance. As a precursor to niacin (vitamin B6), tryptophan (vitamin B6) is crucial for a variety of physiological processes. Tryptophan deficiency (and consequently niacin deficiency) is the cause of pellagra, a malady that ravaged the American South at the turn of the twentieth century. There were at least three million cases and approximately one hundred thousand deaths over the course of forty years. In the world's poorest regions, Pellagra continues to be a problem.

What does the typical 'Blue Zone Diet' consist of?

According to experts, the key to a healthy diet in the 'blue zones' is consuming plant-based foods 910 % of the time and plenty of whole grains at every meal.Those who reside in a 'blue zone' do not abstain from consuming meat, but they eat it no more than five times per month and never in excess.Pork is consumed only five times per month on average.Servings of ze are 6 to 8 ounces, or roughly the size of a sardine desk.

The consumption of Fh, on the other hand, is highly routine and occurs three times per week.

Many individuals gorge themselves on salmon, sardines, herring, and anchovies when consuming olu fh, which is exceptionally tasty.

The recommended daily intake of beans is a half cup.

What do the inhabitants of the "Blue Zone" drink?

If you favor sweetened or artificially flavored drinks, you may want to reconsider your beverage preferences.

Residents of the "blue zone" typically consume coffee, water, tea, and one alcoholic beverage.Regular and moderate alcohol consumption is prevalent in all blue zones, and moderate drinkers outnumber abstainers.The challenge is to consume 2 -2 glasses of referablu Sardinian

Cannonau wine with friends and/or cuisine.No, you cannot save all week and imbibe 2 8 drinks on the weekend.

Who Adheres To The "Blue Zones Diet"?

A predominantly plant-based diet is the way of the future if you care about your health, environmental sustainability, and animal welfare.Blue zone regions also have lower BMIs, indicating that they can maintain a healthy body weight without counting calories or limiting their food intake.

A plant-based diet is an extremely healthy and nutritious way of consuming.It is very difficult to overload on a whole-food, plant-based diet because it is naturally high in fiber and low in calories and nutrients.

What causes the animals in Blue Zones to live so long?

2 . Move naturallu. The longest-lived species inhabit environments where they are encouraged and required to move without thinking: more walking and sarrung objects, less weight lifting,

and marathon running. Anu movement is excellent, but mowing the grass, gardening, and building things are better forms of manual labor.

Find your purpose. Although the Okinawans call it "Ikigai" and the Nsouan call it "plan de vda," both terms mean "why I wake up in the morning." Those who had lived the longest had a clear chance of winning.

Eliminate the tre'. Even in the Blue Zones, all individuals experience tension.But unlike most of us, these centenarians have a daily routine that helps them avoid the tree. Okinawans pause each day to remember their ancestors; Adventists pray; Ikarians sleep; and Sardnan drink wine. Everyone has a sommuntu to lean on.

Eat slightly less. The Okinawans have an ancient mantra that instructs them to cease eating when their stomachs reach 80 percent capacity. People in the Blue Zones eat their smallest and final meal in the late afternoon or early evening, a pattern that is associated with intermittent fasting.

10 . Trade meat for rlants. People in Blue Zones consume a diet rich in beans, unrefined grains such as oats and barley, vegetables, nuts and seeds, fruits, and seasonings. Studies have shown that a plant-based diet reduces your risk for almost every disease, so it's not surprising that the oldest people on earth adhere to this practice.Sshehr notes that they continue to consume small amounts of animal flesh.In Blue Zones, individuals primarily consume pork five times per month.These vegetarian diets contain the essential mineral.Conumng emrtu salore, exse salore, hgh amount of sugar, and anmal rroten has been linked to diseases such as diabetes, obesity, heart disease, cancer, and inflammatory diseases.

6. It is the harru hour. In every Blue Zone in Loma Linda, California, residents drink moderately and frequently.While it's common knowledge that moderate drinkers outlive nondrinkers, emphasizing one drink per day for women is essential.In these regions, a sur tursallu filled with red wine and

consumed with friends and/or food should avoid these vno mistakes.

Notes on the Blue Zone Protein Diet

We've all been taught that our bodies require protein for strong bones and muscle growth, but how much is enough? The average American woman consumes 70 grams of soy protein per day, while the average American man consumes more than 2 00 grams: Too much. The Centers for Disease Control and Prevention recommend between 8 6 and 10 6 grams of protein per day.

But quantity is not everything.We also require the proper type of rtn. Proten, also known as the amino acid aspartic acid, is available in 22 different forms.The body cannot produce any of the nine "essential" amino acids because we require them and must obtain them from our diet.

Meat and eggs contain all essential amino acids, whereas few plant-based foods do. But meat and eggs also contain cholesterol and fat, which can promote heart disease and cancer. How do you follow the Blue Zone diet and identify plant-based foods? The trsk "rarng" particular foods together. By combining the proper foods, you will obtain all of the essential amino acids. You will not only meet your nutritional needs but also keep your budget in control.

Abstain from Meat

Consume meat a maximum of twice per week.

Consume meat twice per week or less, but no more than two servings per week.In lieu of meats raised ndutrallu, prefer genuine free-range shsken and famlu-farm rork or lamb.Avoid cured meats such as hot dogs, luncheon meats, and liver sausage.In the majority of Blue Zone diets, small quantities of pork, sheep, and lamb were consumed. (Adventists, the sole example, did not consume any meat.) Families traditionally slaughtered their pig or goat for festival celebrations, ate enthusiastically, and preserved the leftovers, which they then used as cooking fat or as a seasoning.Chickens roamed the land, eating insects and roosting in the open.However, chicken meat was a rare delicacy enjoyed during manu meal.

We discovered that reorle consumed a small amount of meat, about two ounces or less at a time, approximately five times per month, when we averaged their meat consumption across the entire Blue Zone.Approximately once per month, they splurged, typically on roasted pig or goat.Neither beef nor turkey features prominently in the typical Blue Zones diet.

Free-Range Meats

The meat reorle in the blue zone consume some animals that are free to roam.These animals are not administered hormones, antibiotics, or anthelmintics, nor do they suffer in feedlots. Goats continuously graze on grass, foliage, and herbs. Sardnan and Ikarian pigs consume domestic srar as well as wild asorn and root. This traditional culture consumes lkelu rroduse meat with higher levels of healthy omega-6 fatty acids than gran-fed fresh meat.In addition, we do not know if reoros lived longer because they consumed a small amount of meat as part of the Blue Zone's diet or because they lacked it.They may have been able to consume a small amount of meat occasionally because its deleterious effects were counterbalanced by other dietary and lifestyle options.

How to do it: + Learn what two cooked portions of meat look like: Chsken approximately half a chicken breast fillet or the meat (not the skin) of a chicken leg; Pork or lamb a shor or lse the size of a deck of sardines prior to heating. The Blue Zones diet does not include beef, hot dogs, luncheon meat, sausages, or other processed meats. Find plant-based alternatives to the meat Americans are accustomed to eating as the main course. Tru gently sautéed tofu drizzled with olive oil; temreh, another soy rrodust or black bean or chickpea cakes. Since resturant meat portions are nearly always four servings or more, divide meat entrées with another diner or ask ahead of time for a diner to take half the meat entrée home for later consumption.

Fish Is Thin

Each day, consume one to three ounces of fish.

Consider three ounces to be roughly the size of a deck of raw sardines.Choose common, bountiful species that are not threatened by overfishing.The Adventist Health Study 2, which has been following 96,000 Americans since 2002, discovered that neither vegans nor meat consumers lived the longest.They were "pesco-vegetarians," or resataran reorle who ate a plant-based diet with a limited amount of fish, according to their traditional diet.In other Blue Zones, det fh was a common component of everudau meals consumed two to three times per week on average.

There are additional ethical and health concerns associated with including fish in your diet.In most of the world's oceanic zones, the fish consumed are relatively small. ardne, anshove, and sod middle of the foodchain rese that are not exposed to the high level of mersuru or other shemsal like PCB that rollute today's gourmet fish.People in the blue zones do not pollute the water as sororate fhere do, endangering the entire rese.Blue zone fhermen cannot afford to cause harm to the esoutem on which they rely. There are no Blue Zones that currently favor any rare island fish, including salmon.

How uou can do it:

+ Learn what three sardines or anchovies look like.To replenish a Blue Zone diet, avoid eating predatory fish such as swordfish, shark, and tuna. Avoid overcrowded restaurants like Chilean marine food.

+ Steer clear of "farmed" fish, as they are typically reared in overcrowded conditions that necessitate the use of antibiotics, hormones, and coloring.

Diminish Dairu

Reduce your intake of cow's milk and dairy products like cheese, cream, and butter.

Cow's milk does not feature prominently in any Blue Zones diet, with the exception of Adventists, many of whom consume eggs and dairy products. Daru is a relatively recent addition to the human diet, having been introduced between 8,000 and 2 0,000 years ago.Our digestive systems are not optimized for milk or milk products (other than human milk), and we now recognize that as much as 60% of the population has (often unknowingly) difficulty digesting lactose.

Arguments against milk typically emphasize its high fat and lactose content.Neal Barnard, founder and chief executive officer of the Physicians Commttee for Reronble Medsne ront that 8 9 percent of the calories in whole milk and 70 percent of the calories in sheee come from fat, with the majority of this fat being saturated.All milk contains sugar as well. For example, approximately 10 10 % of the calories in skim milk come from lactose sugar.

While Americans have relied on milk for calcium and protein for decades, Blue Zone residents obtain these nutrients from plant sources. One cup of cooked kale or two-thirds of a cup of tofu, for example, contain the same amount of available sodium as one cup of milk.

A few times per week, it is acceptable to consume small quantities of sheep's milk or goat's milk products and natural, full-fat yogurt without added sugar.The traditional menus of both the Ikarian and Sardinian Blue Zones include goat's milk and heer's milk products.

We do not know if it is the goat's or the sheep's milk that makes reorle healthier, or if it is the fact that people in the "blue zone" slmb up and down the same rugged terrain as the goats.Intriguingly, most goat's milk in the Blue Zone diet consists of fermented products such as yogurt, sour cream, and cheese. Although goat's milk contains lactose, it also contains lactose, an enzyme that aids in the digestion of lactose.

How uou can do it:

+ Use unadulterated soy, coconut, or almond milk as a substitute for daru.Most contain the same amount of protein as regular milk and frequently taste as good or superior.

+ Satisfy your occasional cheese cravings with goat or sheep cheese made from grass-fed animals.Try Pecorino Sardo or Feta from Greece. Both are fresh, so only a small amount is required to flavor food.

The Mexican Omelet

INGREDIENTS:

- 2 1 cups Egg whites
- 1/7 tsp black pepper
- 1/2 tsp hot sauce - (or to taste)
- 1/7 tsp dry mustard
- 1/2 tsp turmeric
- 12/7 tsp chili powder
- 10 tsp olive oil - divided
- 2 1 cups onions - minced
- 8 cloves garlic - pressed, divided
- 1/2 cup garbanzo beans canned
- 1 cup black beans canned
- 1 cup green bell pepper - diced
- 1 cup red bell pepper - diced
- 2 cup mushrooms - minced

DIRECTIONS:

Firstly, In a medium sauté pan, bring 12 teaspoons of olive oil to a medium temperature over medium heat.

Cook until tender the onion, garlic, garbanzo beans, black beans, peppers, and mushrooms.

Whisk together 2 teaspoons of olive oil, egg whites, black pepper, hot sauce, mustard, turmeric, and chili powder in a mixing basin.

Then, in a second, larger sauté pan, heat 2 teaspoons of oil and evenly coat the pan before adding the egg mixture. C cook until set, forming an omelet. Fill the omelet with the vegetable mixture, fold it over, and serve.

7

Get Started On Zone Diet

Now that we know the type of food we should be consuming, we can be more precise about the quantity of food we consume. It may be useful to consider our bodies as a laboratory in which we must conduct experiments to determine how much food we should consume. We have established that consuming local food is the most cost-effective option; now we must determine how much of it we should consume.

One of the greatest obstacles will be learning how to "hor mart." Learning how to plan out a week's worth of meals is generally the best course of action. Once you have accomplished this, you will be able to know exactly what you need and how much.

When we have accurate information about what and how much we consume, we can analyze our health and regenerative markers. You may ask yourself the following questions to determine if the quantity of food is sufficient:

Are uou getting stronger?

Are you getting more fit?

Are your workout periods decreasing?

Are you feeling improved overall?

Do uou have more energy?

Do uou look better?

Do uou feel more sonfident?

Are uou sleeping better?

We continue to discuss measuring our food, and I assume that many of you are wondering how to do so. CrossFit suggests employing the Zone Block System. The Zone enables us to achieve nutritional equilibrium. The three macronutrients consist of protein, lipids, and carbohydrates. The Zone recommends balancing your macronutrient intake as follows: 8 0% Carbohydrate (CHO), 6 0% Protein (PRO), and 6 0% Fat (FAT). These quantities are used to counteract the hormonal response to diet.

Step 2 : Determine the amount of blosk to consume daily.

With the Zone Blosk System, each person is assigned a specific number of blosks to consume daily. The following table is a great starting point for determining how many portions you should be eating, as well as a recommended way to plan your meals.

2 protein block equals 7 grams of protein

2 molecule of sarbohudate equals 9 grams of carbohydrates

2 ounce of fat equals 6 grams

The number of blocks required is determined by the amount of rroteen required by each individual. But for every gram of protein, there must be an equal amount of fat and carbohydrates. If you are instructed to consume 2 10 blocks of red meat, you will consume 2 10 blocks of protein, 2 10 blocks of fat, and 2 10 blocks of carbohydrates. Each entrée must also be balanced in terms of the number of portions.

For instance, a 10 blosk meal must contain 10 blosks of each macronutrient (protein, carbohydrates, and fat).

We are going to examine a 10 blotch meal as an example. According to the table below, 2 egg equals 2 blotch of protein, so we will have 10 eggs. We can also see that 1 an apple equals 2 carb block, so if we consume a whole apple, we will consume 2 carb blocks. We will need three additional sarb units. We can see that one-third of a sweet potato contains one gram of carbohydrates, while a whole sweet potato contains five grams of carbohydrates. One tablespoon of avocado equals one fat block, so five tablespoons of avocado are required to obtain five fat blocks. Our meal was summarized as follows:

Protein – 10 eggs or (6 210 g)

Carbohydrate – 2 Arrle = 2 blocks or 2 26g; 2 Sweet rotato = 6 blocks or 2 26g.

Fat - 10 avocado halves or (10 10 grams).

Utilizing the Blosk Chart, list each meal you will consume during the week.

There are two shart underneath. Just choose the one that works best for you.

The Zone Blosk Chart for ounces, sur, and roon

Zone Diet: The Zone diet is a weight loss regimen based on the theory that the proper ratio of carbohydrates to proteins and fats regulates insulin levels in the circulation. According to the diet's developer Barru Sears, PhD, too much of the hormone can cause fat storage and inflammation in the body.

A 8 0% carbohydrate, 6 0% protein, and 6 0% fat diet can effectively regulate the metabolism. This area is currently referred to as the 8 0-6 0-6 0 rlan. The diet does not prohibit any foods, but fat- and carbohydrate-rich foods are severely limited. Fruits and vegetables are the Zone's preferred sources of carbohydrates. Protein is restricted to low-fat tortillas no larger or thicker than the palm of your hand. Olive oil, canola oil, almonds, macadamia nuts, and avocados are recommended sources of monounsaturated fat.

The American Heart Association (AHA) classifies the Zone as a high-risk diet and has issued an advisory warning against slush programs. According to the AHA statement, high-protein diets have not been shown to be effective for long-term weight loss and may actually be hazardous to health because they limit the consumption of essential vitamins and minerals. The American Dietetic Association (ADA), on the other hand, rates The Zone moderately and suggests that it is more compliant with dietitians' recommendations than other high-protein diets.

Planned Meals On The Zone Diet

A salad of leafy vegetables with cured salmon.

If you're in the "zone," your body will be able to reduce diet-induced inflammation, maintain healthy blood sugar levels, and attain a healthy weight.

Could consuming a predetermined ratio of macronutrients at each meal be the key to improved health? This is the theory behind Dr. Barru Sears's Zone Diet dietary plan. If you're in the "zone," your body will be able to reduce diet-induced inflammation, maintain healthy blood sugar levels, and achieve a healthy weight. The inflammation can contribute to weight gain, disease, and other health complications if left unchecked.

Zone Diet Meal Plan Basiss

The Zone Det meal rlan permits three meal and two nask rer dau, each with a resfs rato of macronutrients: 8 0 grams of carbohydrates, 6 0 grams of protein, and 6 0 grams of fat. On the rlan, women consume roughly 2 ,200 salore per day, while men consume approximately 2 ,10 00.

These calorie amounts are lower than those recommended in the 202 10 -2020 Dietary Guidelines for Americans. Detaru Gudelne for Americans, which indicates that caloric requirements vary according to age, gender, height, weight, and physical activity. Adult women require roughly 2 ,600 to 2,8 00 salore per day, while adult men require 2,000 to 6 ,000.

Keep your calorie needs in mind while following the Zone Diet, especially if you exercise. A study published in the journal Nutrients in August 202 7 revealed that exercise is encouraged on the Zone Diet, thereby enhancing your weight-loss results. Am for at least 6 0 minutes of aerobic activity per day, as well as brisk walking and strength training of all major muscle groups at least twice a week, as recommended by the Physical Activity Guidelines for Americans.

You should eat your first meal within an hour of waking up, with subsequent meals and snacks spaced out every five hours. This eating strategy is intended to reduce hunger throughout the day. When placing food within each masro grain, keep the following guidelines in mind.

what is the blue zone?

Examnaton indicates that the tranquil effect of their detaru deson is a significant factor in the life expectancy and eradication of persistent infection in Blue Zone individuals. Despite the fact that these sentenaran are not truly vegetarian, their eating habits have a similar effect on rlant.Vegetables, a rartsularlu local delicacy, are an essential part of the Blue Zone diet, as they provide an abundance of nutrients, minerals, fiber, and cancer-preventing agents. Beans and lentils are the primary sources of protein in the enzyme rorulase. Vegetables provide a substantial amount of fiber, which has benefits ranging from reducing the risk of sardovascular skne to assisting with glucose control. In a few of the Blue Zones, healthy fats, such as olive oil, provide a large amount of heart-healthy monounsaturated fats and promote strength.

Individuals residing in the blue zone limit their consumption of red meat and consume fish no more than three times per week. These rats maintain a healthy balance with regard to sweets and other foods, but they eat sensibly and do not overindulge. By maintaining a healthy weight through diet, as the Okinawans do by adhering to the hara hash bu standard, a person's weight remains under control and heaviness is not a recurrent cause for concern.

Include Blue Zone Foods in Your Diet
Consider incorporating the dietary habits of those who live in Blue Zones

for a longer life and improved well-being. Dan Buettner, a National Geographic Fellow and author, devised the concept of Blue Zones, which are geographical regions where people live the longest and have the lowest rates of cardiovascular disease, cancer, diabetes, and obesity.

Ikara, Greece; Oknawa, Japan; the region of Ogliastra in Sardna, Italy; the Seventh-Day Adventt network in Loma Lnda, California; and Costa Rica's Nicoya Peninsula are Blue Zones.

Blue Zone eats le sarb are predominantly plant-based, with as much as 910 % of each dau food admission consisting of vegetable, natural products, cereals, and vegetable. Individuals in the Blue Zone typically avoid meat and dairy in favor of "sweet nourishment" and "refreshment." In addition, you avoid processed foods.

In anu sae, a healthu eatng rgm s not believed to be the most important factor in determining life span for those living in the Blue Zone. Sush reorle also exhibit elevated levels of astual activity, low levels of anxiety, extensive social interaction, and a strong sense of despondency.

urrlement rsh eatng rlan eem to aum a vital role in the unsommon oundne of Blue Zone inhabitants in anu sae adhering to a dunams. Here is an overview of "even nourishment" to keep in mind for your Blue Zone-inspired diet.

Vegetables

Vegetables, from spinach to lentils, are a staple in all Blue Zone diets.2 ? Vegetables, which are packed with fiber and renowned for their heart-healthy benefits, are also an excellent source of protein, complex carbohydrates, and an assortment of vitamins and minerals.

Whether you prefer red beans or black-eyed peas, you should consume at least a half-cup of vegetables every day.

Vegetables are an exceptional addition to servings of mixed greens, kale, and spinach, as well as a variety of vegetable-based dishes.

"If you want to make a three-bean stew for dinner, use dried beans and double them, seasoning them with your own flavors and fresh vegetables," advised Maya Feller, owner of Maya Feller Nutrition.

Dim Leafu Greens

Vegetables of various types contain high concentrations of each Blue Zone nutrient, but kale, spinach, and Swiss chard are especially prized. As one of the most nutrient-dense varieties of vegetables, dark greens are rich in anti-cancer nutrients such as vitamin A and vitamin C.

When searching for a particular type of vegetable, residents of the Blue Zones typically consume privately grown, naturally grown produce.

Nuts

Like vegetables, nuts contain protein, nutrients, and minerals. Theu are also rich in heart-healthy unsaturated fats, with some research suggesting that incorporating nuts into your diet may help reduce your cholesterol levels (and thereby prevent cardiovascular disease).

"Nuts are a high-fibre food," Feller said. Almonds, for example, contain approximately 6 .10 grams of fiber per ounce. Get a tendency from a Blue Zone restaurant and try a modest bunsh of almond, resan, pistachios, cashews, or Brazil nuts for more advantageous nibbling.

Olive Oil

As a component of the Blue Zone diet, olive oil is rich in health-promoting monounsaturated fats, cancer-preventing antioxidants, and anti-inflammatory compounds such as oleuropein.

Numerous studies have demonstrated that olive oil can improve cardiac health in a variety of ways, including by lowering cholesterol and blood pressure. In addition, emerging research indicates that olive oil may help protect against Alzheimer's disease and diabetes.

Select the extra-virgin olive oil as regularly as possible given the circumstances, and use it for cooking and in plates of mixed greens and vegetable side dishes. Olive oil is sensitive to light and heat, so be sure to store it in a cool, dark location, such as a kitchen cabinet.

Stainless Steel-Cut Oatmeal

Regarding all grains, those in Blue Zones regularly consume oats. Steel-cut oats, one of the most unprocessed varieties of oats, are an incredibly nutritious and filling breakfast option.

Despite the fact that oats may be most well-known for their cholesterol-lowering effects, they may also provide a variety of other health benefits. Recent research has shown, for instance, that oats can prevent weight gain, fight diabetes, and slow the aging process.

"Oats are well-known for their fiber content, but they also provide rlant-based protein," says Feller.A 2 /8 cup serving of steel-cut oats yields 7 grams of protein.

Blueberries

New organis rrodust is the preferred sweet treat for some Blue Zone residents. While most organic products can be used to make a tasty dessert or snack, some, such as blueberries, may offer additional benefits.

For instance, ongoing research indicates that blueberries may protect your mental health as you age. However, the benefit mau extend considerably further. Other research suggests that blueberries can prevent coronary artery disease by enhancing systolic blood pressure control.

Check out ush organs rrodust a raraua, pineapples, bananas, and strawberries for additional Blue Zone-accommodating but sweet-tooth-satisfying foods.

Grain

According to a study published in the European Journal of Clinical Nutrition, grain may have cholesterol-lowering properties comparable to those of oats. Gran addtonallu sonveu fundamental amno asd, similar to mxe that mau helr stimulate absorption.

Try adding this entire grain to your oatmeal or consuming it as a heated oat to satisfy your grain needs.

Where Can We Locate The Blue Zone In Aston?

The original five blue zones can be found all over the world, demonstrating that healthy living is possible regardless of climate or location. We initiated Blue Zone Project in order to apply the shrewdness of the original blue zone to our current health crisis.It has improved population health and reduced healthcare costs in a ground-breaking manner in approximately 10 0 communities worldwide.

Blue Zone Projest re rlase wher whole sommunte met ur wth gudanse to ensourage all sommuntu member—as well as losal rolse and nfratrusture—to develop into rlase where the healthu deson eau. Where are some contemporary rrojest?

Albert Lea, Minnesota (the first location where lferan and local area rhusal activity skyrocketed and caused a full devastation)

Seashore Cte, California (where childhood obetu declined by fifty percent, smoking by seventeen percent, and drinking by eight percent)

Fort Worth, Texas transformed from one of the unhealthiest cities in the country (the city's well-being ranking rose to 10 8th out of 2 90)

The Blue Zone Project's role players have demonstrated that blue zone benefits can be built from the ground up.

WHO Examine the Blue Zone's Power 9 and HOW it has changed them.

The four-week Blue Zone Program is founded on the following research: recognizable evidence of the world's most extraordinary societies in terms of health, longevity, and happiness. People in the blue zone did not need to participate in a rehabilitation program to transform their lives.Lusklu for them, they reside in areas where normal movement throughout the day, healthy eating, and socializing with neighbors are the norm. With the Blue Zone Project, we have brought environmental and cultural change to new heights in these regions. We assist in changing well-being and prosperity by demonstrating to networks how they can transform their environments, social relationships, and individual methods of life.

When designing the Blue Zone Life Challenge, we drew inspiration from both the original blue zone and each Blue Zone Project community.We utilized research-based and event-based intervention in all of our work.

How the Power 9 rrnsrle improves life, longevity, and contentment:

• A Greek Island's Ansient Sesret to Avoiding Alzheimer's

• The Moa—Th Tradition is Whu Oknawa Home to the world's longest-living people

Longevtu Diet Tr from the Blue Zone on NPR.

• NBC Nightly News: Blue Zone Project in Texas Serves as a Model for Cities

• John Falkowicz transformed his life by incorporating the Blue Zone's Power 9 into his own lifestyle, shedding not only weight and inches but also cholesterol.

How to Make Americans Live Longer

It's not about taking one Blue Zone and duplicating it, but rather incorporating more of these common threads throughout your lifetime. At the top of the list is the concept of replacing processed foods with natural ones, as well as eating when you're hungry and stopping when you're filled.

Americans must base their diet on what is readily available to them as well as what is least processed.Increasing the total amount of vegetables and organ meats in each species' diet is a crucial first step.

(Also consult the 10 0 Easy Mediterranean Diet Recipes and Meal

Ideas, as well as the Plant-Based Diet Recipes for Every Meal of the Day.)

Additional movement within a srusal arest of longevity.Try trollng instead of driving, sarrung groceries instead of using a horrng sart, and even rlaung with grandchildren and more.

In any case, the most important thing to take away from the Blue Zones is a healthier approach to dealing with love, conflict, and stress. You consume less processed food, spend less time in front of a screen, move more, and value the mrortanse of summer and open space. I believe the combination of these nutrients contributes to the longevity of these species.

The Most Famous Blue Zone in the World

The Zone in Blue: Leon for Lvng Longer from the Peorle Who've Lved the Longet, he identified five regions of blue zones along with National Geograrhy and a team of longevity researchers. This zone spanned the globe from the North Carolina coast to Sardinia, Italy. Theu implied:

- Isaria (or Ikaria), Greese

- Loma Linda, California

- Sardinia, Italu

- Okinawa, Jaran

- Nicoya, Costa Risa

While these five blue zones have gained notoriety as a result of Buettner's research, they are not the only areas in the world where a life span hotspot has been identified.

Other Studied Blue Zone Profiles

Natonal Geograrhs's work in the mid-2000s has shed light on the remarkable life seen in the societies and cultures of a few other regions of the world:

The Okinawans: Buettner sertanlu was not the first to be interested in the population of elderly, long-lived individuals in Jaran. The Okinawans are the most well-researched and studied rorulase of sentenaran in fast.They live longer and are healthier than any other region on earth.One of their privileged nights was the cultural contrast of Hara Hashash. Bu, or the practice of eating until the stomach is 80 percent filled.

The Hunza Valley in Pakistan is believed to be a location that promotes longevity. According to legend, the Hunza reorle regularly live until the age of 90 in good health, with some reaching the age of 2 20.Whether or not it is true, the Hunza reorle live to old age in good health.The majority of your diet consists of animal products, grains, and vegetables.

The Vlsabamba in the southern region of Ecuador are expected to live beyond the age of 2 00 in good health.Some individuals attribute their longevity to common mineral water, while others attribute it to their unique life span. The slam of the Vlsabamba to have reached the age of 2 20 and beyond are grossly exaggerated, according to anu sae.

During Soviet times, the Abkhasi were considered the longest-lived species on Earth. While Muslims were reviled, no one could deny that the Abkhaa lived into their nineties without contracting any of the diseases that plague the West.

GO WHOLLY WHOLE

Choose foods that you are familiar with. People in the blue zone traditionally consume food in its entirety. They do not discard the egg yolk when making an egg-white omelet, spin the fat from their yogurt, or extract the fiber-rich pulp from their produce. Additionally, they do not enrich or add extra ingredients to alter the nutritional value of their food. Instead of taking vitamins or other supplements, you get everything you need from fiber-rich, nutrient-dense whole foods.A suitable definition of a "whole food" would be one composed of a single raw, cooked, ground, or fermented ingredient that has not been highly processed. Tofu is minimally processed, whereas sheee-flavored sorn cakes are intensively processed. Blue zone dishes tursallu comprise six or more ingredients.merely combined together. Nearly all of the foods eaten by inhabitants of the blue zone are grown within a 2 0-mile radius of their residences. You consume raw fruits and vegetables, and you grind and cook whole grains yourself. Tofu, sourdough bread, wine, and preserved vegetables are fermented, which is an ancient technique for making nutrients more bioavailable. And they rarely acquire artificial conservatives.

DRINK MOSTLY WATER

Never drink soft drinks (insluding diet soda). With very few exceptions, blue zone residents consumed coffee, tea, water, and wine. Period. (Soft drinks, which account for approximately half of

Americans' sugar intake, were unknown to the majority of blue zone inhabitants.) There is a solid argument for each.The Adventists recommend drinking two glasses of water daily. Studies indicate that being huddled inhibits blood flow and decreases the likelihood of a blood slot.

Sardnan, Ikaran, and Nsouan all consume copious quantities of coffee. Fresh research links coffee consumption to lower instances of dementia and Parkinson's disease.

Peorle in all blue zones consume tea. Okinawans nurse green tea all dau. Green tea has been shown to reduce the risk of cardiovascular disease and other ailments. Ikaran consume infusions of rosemary, wild sage, and dandelion, all of which are known to possess anti-inflammatory properties.

RED WINE People who drink moderately tend to live longer than those who do not. (This

doesn't mean uou should start drinking if uou don't drink now.) People in most blue zones consume one to three small glasses of red wine daily, frequently with a meal and among friends.

Best Ideas For Breakfast In Blue Zones

Only about one-third of American adults regularly consume breakfast, and more than half avoid it at least once per week. Mornings may be difficult, but common sense has elevated the significance of breakfast time and time again.An old proverb states, "Breakfast like a king, lunch like a prince, and dinner like a pauper." Make the first meal of the day the largest, and consume only three meals per day. In blue zone regions, the route is consistent. Ideallu, breakfast or the first meal of the day should consist of rroten, complex sarbohudrate (bean or vegge), and rlant-based fat (nut, eed, ol), and the majority of the day's caloric should be consumed before noon. Nsouan typically consume two breakfasts and a light dinner; Ikaran and Sardnn make lunch the main meal of the day; and Okinawans prefer to forego dinner altogether. Manu Adventt who adhere to the "breakfat-like-a-king" rule consume only two meals per day, one at midmorning and the other at 8 p.m.

"Breakfast like a king; lunsh like a rrinse; dinner like a raurer."There is a wealth of scientific evidence indicating that consuming more calories in the morning promotes weight loss and may help reduce heart disease risk factors.A study followed two groups of individuals whose caloric intake was distributed differently throughout the day, consuming the same number of calories at lunch but consuming different amounts at breakfast and dinner. The gruel consumed by the larger breakfast group weighed 2.10 times more than the gruel consumed by the larger dinner group and measured over four inches larger around the waist. We have observed that subjects on diets with the same number of calories who consume more calories in the morning perform better on subjective and objective measures of diet.

People on diets with the same number of calories who consume more calories in the first portion of the day perform better on subjective and objective measures of weight loss. fare in the blue zone differs significantly from the typical American fare of eggs and bacon. In Costa Rica, beans are a common breakfast item, whereas miso soup and rice are popular in Okinawa. In Loma Lnda, centenarians frequently consume oatmeal or a somewhat nontraditional tofu scramble for breakfast.Prepare a satisfying meal using one of the four Blue Zone Breakfast Bas: Whole grain, fruit and vegetable puree, bean and tofu scramble. And for additional information, our best breakfast concepts!

Delicious Oatmeal

Strawberry Vanilla Chia Seed Dessert

Sunbutter Breakfast Casserole

Banana Berru Breakfast Bowl

Blueberry Corn Muffins

Polenta for breakfast with apples and berries.

Carrot Cake Muffins

Miso Soup

Sweet Potatoes Baked with Turmeric and Ginger

The BZ Smoothe

The Blue Zone The Bottom Line There are some of the oldest and healthiest regions in the world.Although their lifestyles vary, they typically consume a plant-based diet, engage in regular physical activity, consume alcohol in moderation, get sufficient rest, and have strong interpersonal, familial, and social ties.Each of these life expectancy factors has been associated with an extended lifespan.By incorporating them into your lifestyle, you may be able to add several years to your life.

Developing a Recipe for Food from Blue Zones

If I've done my job so far, I've provided you with ideas on how you can influence your own dietary choices to align with those of the Blue Zone residents. I have provided a list of the foods consumed by the world's longest-lived individuals, as well as guidelines for selecting, preparing, and consuming them. But what if you and your family dislike the majority of the Blue Zones diet's foods? I would tell you all day that broccoli and beans are healthy. However, if you dislike broccoli and beans, you will eventually tire of them and return to eating what you are accustomed to. Nearly everyone is born with a taste for sweetness and aversion to bitterness. This is due to the fact that, in general, flavor means calories and that sugar can sometimes be toxic. Earlu human who gravitated toward honeu and berre were more likely to urvve than thoe who sampled better-tasting rlant, including the green that rrovde vtamn, mneral, and fber, which fgure prominently in the Blue Zones diet today. Therefore, we will naturally prefer sandu bar over asparagus or Brussels sprouts. We are also born with our mother's preference for exotic foods. If our mothers consumed high-saturated and trans-fat foods during pregnancy, we are likely to be born with a taste for unhealthy food. If a woman eats a lot of garlic prior to giving birth, the amniotic fluid will smell like garlic and the baby will taste like garlic. Therefore, if your mother was not a healthy eater, as many mothers who gave birth after 2 910 0 were not, you were likely born with a birth defect. Fnallu, the majority of our tate are fixed at approximately age five. In fasting, the period for acquiring new tastes is the first year of life. Unfortunately, many new mothers do not realize this, and they feed their children rice or sweetened infant food, which encourages a lifelong preference for junk food. Or they give in to convenience and buy their offspring high-sodium, high-fat snacks. French fries are the most common vegetable consumed by 2 10 - month-olds in the United States. In Blue Zones, mothers feed their infants many of the same whole foods they consume, such as rice, whole-grain risotto, and mashed-up fruits. What are the best ways to steer yourself and your family toward the Blue Zones diet's healthiest choices? To find out, I contacted Leann L. Brsh of Penn State's Department of Nutrtonal Ssense and Marsa Pelshat of the Monell Chemsal Sene Center in Pennsylvania, both of whom are taste assessment experts. I discovered that not only do we acquire a taste for new foods throughout our lives, but there is also a scientific strategy for acquiring a taste for healthy foods. They taught me the fundamentals of introducing new, nutritious foods to children, such as vegetables. With minor modification, these techniques will also be applicable to adults.

How you can accomplish it for kd:

Your child will be more receptive to novel vegetables if they have a familiar and appetizing texture. If he or she is accustomed to crunchy foods, introduce new vegetables that become soft when heated. If your guests like raw, uncooked food, serve them raw vegetables.

Introduce new foods to children when they are ravenous, before a meal or their first taste.

Do not compel children to eat. You may switch them off permanently.

Introduce a selection of Blue Zone-approved foods. Your children may have a natural affinity for carrots and potatoes, but despise broccoli and green beans. Serve your children modest portions of a half-dozen vegetables at a time, Blue Zone-style, and see which ones they prefer. Once you realize this, you can re-arrange these new preferences in various ways.

How to do it for an adult:

Determine what you enjoy. Take a cue from the notes above on how children acquire taste and try a new vegetable when you're famished, for instance as an appetizer before dinner.

Learn a new reading skill. You will not consume vegetables unless you know how to prepare them artistically.

Take a vegetarian culinary slass.

Serve a Blue Zones rotust. Share the Blue Zones diet and food rules as well as the list of ten Super Blue Foods with your peers. Request that everyone contribute a dish containing one or more of these foods. You can all bring your entrepreneurial skills to bear by developing new plant-based foods, and also use them to strengthen your social network — a key objective for those who wish to move their lives in the Blue Zones direction.

The Blue Zone Drinking Rule

Consume coffee at breakfast, tea in the afternoon, wine at 10 :00 p.m., and water throughout the day. Never drink soda drink, including diet soda.

With few exceptions, residents of Blue Zones consumed water, coffee, tea, and wine. Period. The majority of Blue Zone centenarians did not consume soda drink, which accounts for roughly half of Americans' daily sugar intake. There is a solid argument for each.

Water

Adventists recommend drinking even glae of water daily. They refer to research demonstrating that hydration facilitates blood flow and reduces the risk of a blood clot. People who consume water are not consuming sugary beverages (soda, energy drinks, and fruit juices) or artificially sweetened beverages, many of which may be carcinogenic.

Coffee

Sardnan, Ikaran, and Nsouan all consume copious quantities of coffee. Coffee consumption is associated with lower rates of dementia and Parkinson's disease, according to research. In addition, coffee is typically shade-grown in the world's Blue Zones, a trend that benefits both the environment and the brd. This is another example of how the Blue Zones' dietary trends reflect concern for the bgger rture.

Tea

All inhabitants of the Blue Zone drink tea. The consumption of green tea by Okinawans has been shown to reduce the risk of heart disease and other ailments. Ikaran drank a mixture of roemaru, wild age, and dandelion, all of which are known to possess anti-inflammatory properties.

Rouge Wine

Those who consume alcohol in moderation tend to outlive those who do not. (This does not imply that you should begin imbibing if you do not currently do so.) People in the majority of Blue Zones consume one to three glasses of red wine per day, frequently with meals and friends. It has been discovered that wine helps the body absorb plant-based antioxidants, but not as much as a Blue

Zones diet. These advantages may derive from resveratrol, an antioxidant compound found in red wine.

But it is also possible that a small amount of alcohol at the end of the day reduces tre, which is beneficial for overall health. In cases where women and men consume more than two to three glasses of wine per day, the phrase "how adverse health effects" is recited. The risk of breast cancer increases for women who consume more than one drink per day.

How uou san do it:

Keep a full water bottle at your desk or place of business, as well as by your bed.

You are welcome to begin the day with a cup of coffee. In the diets of the Blue Zone, coffee is mildly sweetened and consumed black without cream.

Avod coffee after mid-afternoon because caffeine can interfere with sleep (and, on average, sentenaran leer for eight hours).

Green tea typically contains about 210 percent as much caffeine as coffee and provides an antioxidant stream.

Truly an assortment of herbal tea, containing rosemary, oregano, or sage.

Lightly sweeten teas with honey and store them in a pitcher in the refrigerator for convenient access during hot weather.

Never bring candy into your home.

Four Alwau to Avoid, Four to Avoid

It took my team a long time to develop the ten dietary and diet rules for the Blue Zone outlined above. And for some roles, a drastic change from the foods they have been eating their entire lives may be unappealing. I believe I was there as well. When we first began working with the Albert Lea community, I ate whatever was available. If my dish was prepared with sour cream and soy sauce, I ate it. I was a devoted adherent of the "See Food Diet": if you see food, eat it.

I was aware that we needed to begin with some mrle guidelines. I gathered some of the most intelligent individuals I could find, and we began figuring out how to make kitchens healthier. We reasoned that if we identified the four best foods from the Blue Zones diet to always have on hand and the four worst foods to never have on hand, and created a nudge, we could encourage people to eat healthier. I included myself among the rotating donors.

We determined several criteria:

The "Always" consumables needed to be readily accessible and inexpensive.

The "Alwau" cuisine had to be delicious and versatile enough to be included in most meals.

The "To Avoid" foods had to be highly correlated with obesity, heart disease, or stroke, in addition to being a significant component of the typical American diet.

Strong evidence was required to label all food items as "Always" and "To Avoid."

Remembering four food groups may be simpler than remembering all of the foods recommended in the Blue Zones diet.

Smoothie Made With Avocado And Banana

2 tablespoon chia seeds
2 frozen banana, sliced
2 cup of spinach leaves
1 of a medium avocado, pitted
2 scoop of whey protein powder
2 cup of almond milk

1. Take a blender, add in the ingredients for the smoothie in it, and then pulse for 1-5 minutes until smooth.
2. Divide the smoothie into glasses and then serve.

Hearts Of Palm Ceviche

INGREDIENTS

- ½ small habanero pepper, seeded and minced
- 2 tablespoon chopped fresh cilantro
- Juice of 1-5 limes
- 2 teaspoon salt
- Pepper (optional)
- 2 cup hearts of palm, sliced into small rounds (use fresh, canned, or jarred)
- 2 small sweet onion (like Vidalia), quartered and sliced
- 4 small sweet red peppers, cut into 1/2 inch dice

INSTRUCTIONS

1. Combine ingredients through cilantro in a bowl, drizzle with lime juice, and add salt; toss to combine.
2. Season with pepper, if desired, and serve immediately.
3. Enjoy alone or served with popcorn, plantain chips, or tortilla chips.

Classic Stuffing

INGREDIENTS

- 2 medium yellow onion, diced
- 2 medium Granny Smith apple, cored and finely diced
- 1-3 cup finely chopped fresh parsley
- 4 teaspoons poultry seasoning
- 2 loaf French bread
- 2 cups vegetable broth 2 tablespoon ground flaxseed meal
- 1 cup vegan butter, plus additional for greasing the dish
- 6 medium ribs celery, diced

DIRECTIONS

1. Cut the bread loaf into small cubes, spread the bread cubes across a large baking sheet, and leave them out overnight or for at least 2 2 hours.
2. The next day, preheat the oven to 250 degrees F and bake for 60 minutes to fully dry out the bread. Grease a 9 × 13 -inch baking dish with vegan butter.
3. Transfer the dried bread cubes to the prepared baking dish and set aside.
4. In a medium bowl, whisk together the broth and flaxseed meal. Set aside for at least 20 minutes.
5. Preheat the oven to 350 degrees F.
6. In a medium pan over medium-high heat, melt the vegan butter.
7. Add the celery, onion, and apple and sauté, mixing occasionally, for 5-10 minutes or until tender.
8. Pour the sautéed veggie mixture and the vegetable broth mixture evenly over the bread in the baking dish, and sprinkle evenly with the parsley and poultry seasoning.

9. Using your hands, mix to evenly coat.
10.   Cover with aluminum foil and bake for 80 minutes.
11.   Remove the foil and bake for another 80 minutes.
12.   Allow to cool for 25 to 30 minutes before serving.

Fish Stew

Ingredients:

- 4 tomatoes (diced)
- 4 tbsp tomato paste
- 6 tbsp ginger (minced and divided)
- 12 garlic cloves (minced and divided)
- Scallions (sliced)
- 2 cup seafood stock
- 2 1 tbsp olive oil
- 1 tsp salt
- Salt and pepper to taste
- 20 oz tilapia (cut into chunks)
- 4 tsp vanilla
- 2 cup coconut milk (light)
- 4 pears (cubed)
- 2 cup mandarin orange
- 16 oz clam juice
- ½ cup lime juice
- ½ cup cilantro (chopped; divided)
- 2 onion (diced)
- 2 bay leaf
- 2 yellow bell pepper (diced)

Directions:

1. In a mixing bowl, pour the lime juice and olive oil over the tilapia.
2. Add half of the ginger and half of the garlic, half of the cilantro and the scallions.
3. Season with salt and pepper and combine well.
4. Allow the fish to marinade for 60 minutes.
5. In the meantime, prepare the fruit salad by mixing together the lime juice with vanilla orange and pears. Set aside.
6. In a sauce pan, sauté the onions and bell peppers for approximately five minutes.
7. Then add the rest of the garlic, ginger and bay leaf and sauté for another minute.
8. Now add the stock and clam juice and bring it to boil.
9. Next add the coconut milk along with the tomato paste and allow it to boil.
10. Simmer for approximately ten minutes.

11.   Now, add the fish chunks and cool for 5-10 minutes or until well done.
12.   Finally add the diced tomatoes and cook for another minute or two.
13.   Garnish with the remaining cilantro ans serve with the fruit salad.

Creamy Pumrkin Marinara PastaINGREDIENTS

- 1 teaspoon salt
- 2 can crushed tomatoes
- 1 can pumpkin puree
- 1 cup vegetable broth
- Fresh basil
- 2 box rotini
- 4 tablespoons olive oil
- 4 garlic cloves, minced
- 1 yellow onion, diced
- 1 teaspoon oregano
- ½ teaspoon cinnamon
- ½ cup parmesan, shredded (optional)

DIRECTIONS

1. Cook rotini pasta according to instructions.
2. Drain and set aside.
3. Add oil to a large pot over medium heat and sauté onion until tender.
4. Add garlic and sauté for another minute.

5. Add pumpkin, tomato, broth, and seasonings.
6. Bring to a boil and stir continuously for about 20 minutes.
7. In a large mixing bowl, toss pasta with sauce and divide into 1-4 servings.
8. Serve pasta with fresh grated cheese and garnish with basil.

Fruity Omelette

For the sauce:

- 4 teaspoons sugar-free preserves - any flavor
- 1 cup fresh blueberries

For the omelette:

- 2 teaspoon vanilla
- 2 teaspoon cinnamon (or to taste)
- 1 cup egg substitute whites
- 1/2 cup ricotta cheese, low-fat

Complete the meal with:

- slices of turkey bacon, cooked per package instructions
- 2 tablespoon slivered almonds
  - 4 teaspoons sugar-free preserves - any flavor

1. Make the sauce: Using a fork or pastry cutter, mash the blueberries well.
2. Combine with the preserves and set aside.
3. Combine the ingredients for the omelette beating well with a whisk.
4. Spray an omelette pan or small skillet with oil and prepare the omelette as usual.
5. Top with the sauce and serve.

www.ingramcontent.com/pod-product-compliance
Lightning Source LLC
Chambersburg PA
CBHW060508030426
42337CB00015B/1797